The Smart & Easy Guide To Skin Care: The Best Natural, Organic, Herbal, DIY, And Over The Counter Skincare Treatments & Recipes For Healthier Skin & Anti Aging Remedies

Elizabeth White

I0415626

Legal Stuff

DISCLAIMER

THIS BOOK IS NOT DESIGNED TO, AND DOES NOT, PROVIDE MEDICAL ADVICE. ALL CONTENT ("CONTENT"), INCLUDING TEXT, GRAPHICS, IMAGES AND INFORMATION AVAILABLE IN OR THROUGH THIS BOOK ARE FOR GENERAL INFORMATIONAL PURPOSES ONLY.

THE CONTENT IS NOT INTENDED TO BE A SUBSTITUTE FOR PROFESSIONAL MEDICAL ADVICE, DIAGNOSIS OR TREATMENT. NEVER DISREGARD PROFESSIONAL MEDICAL ADVICE, OR DELAY IN SEEKING IT, BECAUSE OF SOMETHING YOU HAVE READ ON THIS BOOK. NEVER RELY ON INFORMATION ON THIS BOOK IN PLACE OF SEEKING PROFESSIONAL MEDICAL ADVICE.

THE AUTHOR, PUBLISHER AND ALL AFFILIATED PARTIES ARE NOT RESPONSIBLE OR LIABLE FOR ANY ADVICE, COURSE OF TREATMENT, DIAGNOSIS OR ANY OTHER INFORMATION, SERVICES OR PRODUCTS THAT YOU OBTAIN THROUGH THIS SITE. YOU ARE ENCOURAGED TO CONFER WITH YOUR DOCTOR WITH REGARD TO INFORMATION CONTAINED IN OR THROUGH THIS BOOK. AFTER READING THIS BOOK, YOU ARE ENCOURAGED TO REVIEW THE INFORMATION CAREFULLY WITH YOUR PROFESSIONAL HEALTHCARE PROVIDER.

LIMITATION OF LIABILITY

Table of Contents

Why Its Important to Care for Your Skin

When looking at the majority of marketing companies out there, and those companies which provide products to the consumer market, they look at the packaging as being just as important as the product itself. With this idea in mind, a person will want to take the same types of thoughts when it comes to their personal appearance. Your skin is just as important as what you have on the inside. There are many people who realize that having a routine for their skin is important. This can be seen from the wide range of skin care products on the market. Most people think that a person who has good skin is a person that looks good, yet there is more than looks associated with good skin.

Those who have good skin are going to have higher self-esteem in most cases. A person who knows their skin looks good is the person that is going to feel more energetic and ready to take on the world. These people tend to work faster and harder since they feel so good about themselves. Those who have good skin often have their genes to compliment, yet the products that a person uses is going to have a profound effect on the health of skin.

In addition to being more energetic and having a good self-esteem, those who have good skin are often reported to have people be friendlier towards them. Other people tend to respect someone who looks good, meaning if their skin is at its best. Those who are around you are going to be envious of your skin, and they may even ask you about your skin care routine in order to copy the results you are getting. It is up to you, whether you choose to divulge this information or not.

Those who do not take the time to ensure their skin is as healthy as it can be are often those who feel as though they are getting treated poorly in life. Those who have bad skin often look as though they are lifeless and dull. Because of this, the person may have a harder time staying on task, or even being friendly with those that they met. The aging process can start much earlier for those who have bad skin as they are going to look older than their years.

With all this in mind, it is imperative that a person has a skin care routine that is going to work for them. The good news is that achieving good skin is not hard. There are several products on the market that are meant to help suit every type of skin that is out there. In order to start this process, a person must know how these products are classified to know which product is going to work the best for you.

Products are classified in areas such as:

- Skin Type: These products are going to be for a certain skin type such as oily, dry skin, sensitive skin, or combination skin.

- Use: Many products are categorized based on how they should be used. For example, they may be considered cleansers, moisturizers, toners, or for exfoliation.

- Treatment: Several products are going to be catered towards the problem a person may have with their skin. For example, products that are meant to diminish fine lines and wrinkles, those which are meant to help with acne and those which are meant to help reduce stretch marks.

- Ingredients: Several products are going to be classified according to the types of ingredients that are found in the product. These categories can be all natural, organic, cosmetic and so forth.

Aside from understanding what type of classification a product is, the person does need to realize that the skin routine they adopt is just as important as the classification of the product.

The Routine for Skin

Knowing how important it is to care for your skin is a great start to building up a good skin routine. However, the routine of a person is going to vary from individual to individual. There are those who believe they have to visit a professional every day in order to have the skin they have. While others are dependent upon their own products they buy for their skin. Still, there are others who believe they should only pay attention to their skin once every few months. The good thing to remember is that a personal skin care routine is not going to be expensive, and it is easy to put into your busy schedule. The rewards that you will reap from doing this are too huge to pass up.

The routine that you have for your skin is a procedure that will be repeated each day. In order to start developing the routine you first need to know what your skin type is. The skin type can be oily, dry, sensitive, normal, combination or acne prone. Most people will find that they can take a normal skin care routine and adopt this to fit their personal needs. The personal skin care routine for a normal skinned person will consist of Cleansing, Exfoliating, Moisturizing and applying Sunscreen.

The cleansing phase is meant to clean the face of oils, dirts and the like that have made their home in your skin. Most cleansers are going to contain oil, water and other agents that are meant to dig deep into the skin and pull out the impurities found there. There are several cleansing products on the market, meaning that you may have to try a couple before you find the one that best suits your skin. However, you should always use a cleanser that is soap free as soap can be drying and irritating to skin. Also remember to use luke warm water when washing your skin to avoid further damage to the skin.

Exfoliating the skin is the process of removing dead skin cells that could clog the pores of the skin. This usually follows the cleansing phase of the skin care routine. However, this is not something that a person has to do everyday. In fact, most people recommend doing this only 3-5 times per week, or adjusting this to meet your needs. The weather and your skin type are all going to affect how much you have do this in order to keep your skin healthy.

Moisturizing your skin is vital, even for those who feel they have oily skin naturally. Moisturizers not only help to keep moisture in the skin but also allow moisture from the air to get into the skin whenever this is needed. You will need to use a small amount of moisturizer to avoid causing more problems to your skin. For the best results, a person should apply the moisturizer when their skin is still damp.

The use of sunscreen is recommended for every day of the year. Luckily, many moisturizers put this into their lotion in order to give the person an added benefit of using it. You will want to use this in the morning before you go outside, even if the Sun is not shining that day.

You are going to have to experiment with many products and the amount of these products to find what works best for you. If you find that you cannot perfect this routine, it may be time to visit a dermatologist to find if you have a special skin condition that may be in need of special skin products.

Skin Care Basics

The older generation seemed to have it much easier when it came to skin care. They washed their skin with soap and went about their day. However, research and science has proven that this is not the best method. Nowadays, there are tons of skin products on the market that makes it hard for a person to know just where they should turn for their product and skin care routine. There are lotions, ointments, and masks in every skin care aisle within every store, making it hard for a person to know what to choose. Yet, in order for a person to make a decision they do need to know information on the types of products that are out there.

Stress, sun damage, pollution, and poor diets are reflected on the skin of every woman that walks around. Due to the number of damage skin can go through, there is a need for products that are going to counteract these problems. Lotion is one of the basics of any skin care routine. Lotions are vital because they help the skin to stay moisturized. When skin is properly hydrated, it is going to be luminous. When the skin is dehydrated, it is going to show. With this being said, lotion needs to be used at least twice a day to reap the full benefits.

Lotions come in various types meant to be used on different parts of the body. You should always use a lotion that is hypoallergenic in order to avoid clogging your pores. Lotion that is used for the face is often called moisturizers while lotion for the entire body is referred to as 'body lotion'. Body lotions are not meant to be used on the face as they are thicker and can cause the pores to clog. Knowing your skin type can make it easier to find the best lotion since you will know just how much moisturizer your skin is going to need.

Ointments are often for problems with the skin such as having rashes or eczema. There are also specialty creams that may be called ointments that are meant to do things such as reduce wrinkles or lines. Most ointments are meant to be used in the eye area as they are going to be a bit gentler, and they can have a great effect on the healthy glow of the skin.

Skin masks are meant to be something that is used once or twice a week. These are often seen as the best way to give your skin a fresh look a few times per week. There are many different ingredients that make up a skin masks. For example, there are those that are meant to smooth the skin, hydrate the skin, tighten the pores, and those that are meant to help with acne. All skin masks are going to make your skin appear smoother. Once you apply a mask you will feel it start to tighten the skin as it dries. Most masks are going to require that you wait for ten or fifteen minutes then rinse this off the face. You will want to use either a washcloth or water alone, depending on the sensitivity of your skin.

There are full body masks that are meant to help your entire body tighten and feel refreshed. When getting a full body mask, the person should be sure they stay hydrated. These masks tend to pull the water from your body and can make a person very thirsty.

Through arming yourself with the knowledge about the types of products that are out there, you are going to get the skin that you have always desired. Hydration is the main key to getting skin that is glowing and healthy, meaning that you should always drink water to hydrate from the inside to the outside.

Tips for Skin Care

For those who want to have healthy skin there are ten tips that they can use and integrate into their beauty routine in order to get the skin that they want. These ten tips are just a slice of what a person can do in order to maximize the health of their skin. However, they are some of the most important things that a person can do.

1. Know your skin type. This cannot be emphasized enough as the products that you use are geared towards your skin type. If you do not know your skin type you cannot possibly get the nutrients that your skin needs in order to flourish.

2. Drink water, and this does not mean that you should limit yourself to just a few sips a day. The best advice that someone can take is to drink the recommended amount of water everyday. This is going to keep your skin healthy because it provides the essential moisturizing that you need from the inside out.

3. Always cleanse your skin regularly, which is usually one to two times per day depending on your skin type. This is going to help to get rid of elements that could cause your skin to get oilier or cause acne. Always remember to use warm water for cleansing as using hot or cold water can cause more damage to your skin.

4. Be gentle with your skin, even when cleansing. Your skin is delicate and the more that your scrub in an effort to remove the dirt and debris from the skin, the more you are damaging your skin.

5. Always ensure that your skin is moist because dry skin can be damaged even more by the elements that a person is exposed to each day. When using a moisturizer, remember that it is going to work best if the skin is damp, rather than dry.

6. Do not use soap on your face, as soap is a drying agent and can cause your skin to become more dry and irritated. Soap is only meant to be used on the skin below your neck.

7. Always wear sunscreen, even if the day is cloudy. Harmful sunrays can be damaging to the skin even if you do not see the sun throughout the day. It is the rays from the sun that are linked to the cause of skin cancer, thus you should always use sunscreen.

8. Exercise and maintain a good sleep schedule. Your skin looks its best when you are at your best on the inside. Lack of exercise is the leading cause of skin sagging, while not having enough sleep can cause wrinkles and dark circles in the skin, dyspeptical under the eyes. In addition, when you exercise and get the right amount of sleep, you are beating stress which can cause damage to the skin.

9. Always treat any problems with your skin with care. For example, if you have acne, then use products that are still gentle on the skin in order to combat the problem. The best piece of advice is to see a dermatologist about the skin problems you may be having, as the medical professional is going to know what to do to minimize damage, while also treating the problem.

10. Do not let stress get you down, meaning that take a little time out of each day for yourself in order to relax. Do whatever it is that is going to help you get back on the right level, as your skin will be rewarded for doing this.

Common Skin Conditions: How to Care for These

Whenever you have a condition with your skin that is causing it to be less than stellar, you want results that are going to give you the healthy skin that you crave. With this being said, there are treatments for just about every skin condition on the market. It is vital that a person choose the treatment that is best suited for their skin type in order to avoid having any problems stemming from treatment. The good news is that the majority of skin problems a person has can be prevented through having a skin care routine that is going to prevent problems from growing. This is often referred to as preventive skin care or proactive skin care. However, those who have a skin care routine will find that there are certain skin problems that will still occur, thus meaning that the person needs to seek additional treatment.

One of the most common problems that are found with the skin is acne. The idea is to control acne and prevent this acne from getting worse. In order to do this you should consider wearing light clothes that are not too confining, since the more tight a piece of clothing is the more sweat that is being trapped in the pores. You should also not touch the blemish constantly, as the oils on the hands can cause the infection to get worse, and prolong the stay of the acne. You will still want to be gentle with your skin care routine in order to avoid aggravating the acne that you do have. You can purchase an over the counter product that is meant to help control and prevent acne in order to get the skin you want.

Dry skin is another type of skin ailment that is regularly reported, and it is easily fixed. The person will want to have a moisturizer that they can use, but they also need to know how to use this in order to maximize the benefits of using it. The best route is to apply the moisturizer while the skin is still damp. You will want to avoid not applying enough moisturizer and applying too much as this can make the problem worse. If you have not seen any dramatic results within three to four weeks, then a visit to the dermatologist may be warranted.

Sun spots or brown spots are what happens to the skin when it has been exposed to the rays of the sun. In order to avoid this problem getting worse, always remember to wear sunscreen that is at least 15 SPF. You may also find it helpful to wear clothing that is going to cover the areas in which brown spots are appearing to protect it even more from the rays of the sun.

Keep in mind that if you are using over the counter products and these are not working that you may have to go to a professional to find the best product. The dermatologist that a person sees is going to take into consideration their problem, the products they have used and their skin routine to know whether the person may need some type of pharmaceutical grade product to work on their skin.

Skin Care for Oily Skin

Oily skin is common for many people and it can be a huge game changer for those who are trying to get healthy and glowing skin. Oily skin is caused by too much oil in the skin, this is the over production of sebum. The more oily the skin, the more likely the person is to find their pores clogged, causing acne. Other people will find that simply having oily skin makes their skin look less healthy since it does cause a sheen to develop over the skin and it makes the skin look dirty.

When looking for a skin care routine for oily skin the main objective is to remove the excessive oil from the skin. You do not want to remove all of it, because this can lead to the skin becoming excessively dry. In order to start this process, it is imperative that the person uses a cleanser that is designed for oily skin. The best products are those that have a salicylic acid in them that is meant to combat the extra oil the skin is producing. Always be sure that you check that the product is oil free, which should not be a problem when looking at products for oily skin.

For those who have extremely oily skin they are going to be able to use a product that is alcohol based, since they can ensure their skin is not going to dry out from the use of this. However, keep in mind that the more alcohol you use on your skin, the more damage that you could be doing.

Even though you have oily skin, you will still need a moisturizer, however, this needs to be a milk moisturizer. You will want a lotion that is oil free, wax free and free of lipids since these ingredients can cause skin to become even oilier.

With all the skin products on the market, you may have to try out many before you find something that works. If you find that no over the counter product is helping at all, then you may need to talk with a dermatologist to figure out the best plan for your skin. There are many products on the market that are stronger, yet require a prescription since they contain retinoid and sulfur ingredients.

Skin Care for Dry Skin

Dry skin is something that must not be ignored by those who have this. The drier the skin is the more cracking that the outer layer of skin is going to experience, which can lead to a bad appearance. Dry skin is caused by many things such as a dry climate, hormonal changes, or even doing too much to your skin with your care routine. Many people will find that they naturally have dry skin. The good news is that treating dry skin is not difficult at all.

In order to combat dry skin always remember to moisturize. There are those moisturizers that are meant to combat the dryness by sealing in the moisture that the skin naturally has. These types of moisturizers are readily available at almost any store and are fairly inexpensive. The other way that moisturizers can help a person is through actually taking moisture from the environment and putting this into the skin.

Since moisturizing is such a huge issue with dry skin, it is important that the person realize that they need to apply their moisturizer appropriately. This means doing this when the skin is still damp and the moisturizing lotion or cream is not full of products that could cause harm.

There are several natural products on the market that utilize no chemicals or other products that are manufactured in order to treat the skin that is dry. Thus, this is something that a person will want to consider finding. Never should a person use any type of product on dry skin that contains alcohol or detergents as this can actually cause the skin to become worse.

Combination Skin Care

There are several people who have a problem with certain areas of their skin being dry while other areas are riddled with moisture. For a person who has combination skin, it may seem as though they can never get the skin they want since they are dealing with two totally opposite problems. For the most part, the T-zone of the face is where the person will experience the most oil.

If you are uncertain as to whether you have combination skin, there are many ways in which you can determine this. For example, after washing your face are there certain areas of the skin that seem tight and may even be rough to the touch? Secondly, the appearance of your skin will include patches that are shiny with oil, while other parts of the skin are dry and dim.

Caring for combination skin can seem like a huge hassle to those who have this problem. There are hinges that you can do in order to avoid feeling as though your problem skin is taking over.

1. Cleanse your skin every day, and you may find that using a mild cleaner is the best option. For those with combination skin it is best that they cleanse once at night before bed and once in the morning before starting your day.

2. Use a moisturizer that is going to identify what areas of the skin need more moisture and what areas do not. You may find that you have to use two different moisturizers to combat the two problems that you have.

The ultimate goal for combination skin is to make the skin as normal as possible, meaning that you want the dry and oil areas to mix to the point of perfection. Products that contain hydroxyl acids or retinols are great for people with combination skin as they do help to achieve a normal look. The reason that these products work so well is because they help with skin cell regeneration. They remove the top layer of skin that is too oily or too dry and expose the skin beneath that is healthier. The second layer of skin is more likely to absorb moisture better to help combat the 'tight' feel to skin that many people complain about when they have dry skin in certain areas. You do need to make a note that once you start using these products that you will have to continue to use them in order to keep your skin looking great. These are not products that are meant to correct the problem once and be done with these.

The shine that most combination skin has is annoying for many people. This is the other aspect that the person will need to contend with. Makeup that is designed to be oil absorbing is a great way to ensure that the skin looks great all day long. You will find that this makeup will greatly benefit your T-zone, since this is the area that sees the most oil on many people.

Those with combination skin are often embarrassed and annoyed with their skin. However, you can make changes that are going to make your skin appear more natural and healthy. The key is to use the products as they are meant to be used for combination skin and avoid making the dry areas more dry and the oily areas oilier.

Skin Care for Acne

Acne is a problem that most people have at least one time in their life, and many people live with this for several years. Acne is defined as having a disease associated with the hair and oil glands. Acne involves pimples, reddish tint to the skin, black/white heads and cysts. Facial acne is something that can cause embarrassment and spoil a person's appearance to the point in which they feel very uncomfortable. Acne is a problem that a person should try to alleviate, and they can with the proper skin care routine.

Caring for acne should really start before the acne is seen, as it is easier to alleviate the problem before it gets out of hand. In fact, skin care for acne is more about preventing acne rather than treating the current acne a person is dealing with. To start the skin care routine for acne, the skin needs to be cleansed in order to help alleviate the oil and dirt in pores that is causing the problem. Cleansing the face and taking a shower at night can be a huge help in relieving the acne problem, especially for those who live in climates that are hot and humid. The reason for this is that it allows the sweat that has been building on the skin to be removed at night before the person is asleep and the sweat is able to build into the pores more.

On top of this, the person needs to wear clean clothes and sleep on sheets and pillows that are clean. Oil can seep into clothing and bed linens which can then transfer back onto the body causing more problem. Tight clothing is also an issue for those who deal with acne, as this does not allow the skin to breath. Cotton clothing is recommended for those who are trying to stop acne before it starts.

The cleansers that you use on your skin need to be water based and be free of oils and soaps as these can cause the skin to become even more irritated. For women, they should also remove their makeup before going to sleep at night, as this can cause more oil to build up into the skin which in turns causes more acne.

If you are already dealing with acne, be sure that you do not touch the acne or squeeze this as this can lead to scars on the skin. Gentle cleansing of the affected area is going to help to rid the acne before it gets worse. You can also use an over the counter medication to treat the acne that is already on the skin, as there are several over the counter acne products to choose from. If the acne does not respond to a new care routine or medication then it is best to seek a professional's help in determining what you can do to rid your skin of acne.

Skin Care for Sensitive Skin

Sensitive skin means that the person's skin is unable to tolerate conditions that are considered tolerable for many other people. In turn, the skin can easily become irritated, itch or the like due to the conditions that it is being exposed to. It can make it hard for a person to do anything with their skin, as they are never sure as to what the end results will be. There are many products on the market that are meant to be used for those with sensitive skin and have ingredients that are gentler. No skin type if going to respond well to harsh ingredients, however, sensitive skin is going to respond negatively at the beginning of such treatment. There are several tips that a person can use if they have sensitive skin which is going to help them to have healthy skin, and avoid the irritation that comes with having skin that is sensitive.

1. Only use products that are designed for sensitive skin and make sure that you read the directions on how to use this in order to avoid any irritation. With this in mind, you should make sure that the product you choose has minimum ingredients and additives that could cause a problem.

2. Never should you use toners as these are based with alcohol, a huge problem for those with sensitive skin.

3. You should protect your skin whenever possible in order to avoid irritating this. For example, you may want to wear gloves when doing the dishes or laundry.

4. Always wear sunscreen before going out in the sun as sensitive skin has a tendency to burn easier. In fact, you may want to consider a higher SPF when dealing with sensitive skin.

5. Always wear clothing that is going to cover you from irritants in the environment.

6. A moisturizer that is noncomedogenic is best for sensitive skin, yet you will not see that this type of moisturizer is labeled towards those with sensitive skin.

7. Use a cleanser that is free of soap and alcohol as this can cause problems. And always cleanse your skin when you have been exposed to irritants, such as being outdoors.

8. Exfoliating needs to be done with care, and many people with sensitive skin are going to find that this needs to be avoided altogether.

9. Those who wear makeup will not want to wear this for very long, because this can cause more irritation.

Though it is hard to deal with sensitive skin it can be done. The main aspect to keep in mind is that you have to be gentler with this type of skin to avoid problems and unsightly blemishes.

Caring for Your Facial Skin

The skin on your face needs to be dealt with in a cleaner manner than the rest of your body. The routine that a person has for their face is much different than what they do for the rest of their body. There are four basic steps for facial skin which are cleansing, toning, exfoliating and moisturizing the face.

The first step with facial skin is to cleanse the skin appropriately. This is going to remove any irritants or pollutants that could cause more problems for your skin. Most professionals recommend using a cleansing cream or lotion and delicately applying this to the face with a cotton ball. After applying this, wipe it clean with a soft cotton or tissue, however, do not rub the skin as this can cause irritation. You should clean your face at least two times a day, usually once in the morning and once at night. Cleansers that are water based are usually the best bet for facial skin.

Toning is not something that everyone has to do, yet most people include this in their daily skin routine. Toning is basically meant to help remove any dirt or excess cleaner that is left behind. With this being said, those who properly cleanse their face can avoid this step. Those who do want to tone may find it best for their skin to only do this on days in which they have seen a lot of irritants to their skin, such as being outside and sweating throughout the day.

Exfoliating is also an optional step for many people, though they are not going to want to do this everyday. Once or twice a week is usually the maximum for when a person should do this. They are going to find that exfoliation basically removes the dead skin cells to help the skin appear brighter and healthier. However, when you use this more frequently than what is suggested, this can damage the skin to the point in which the person may become irritated.

Moisturizing is a step that everyone should be doing. This is one of those steps that a person really cannot avoid if they want healthy skin. Even if your skin is oily, it does need a moisturizer used on it. It is best to apply your moisturizer when your skin is damp as it absorbs better.

The following are some tips that can help aid in caring for your face:

1. Use a make up remover for makeup instead of just rubbing this off with water.

2. Choose your facial products based on your skin type.

3. Try out a new product on a small piece of skin such as behind the ears to see how you are going to react.

4. Never rub the skin as this can cause irritation.

5. Always wear sunscreen.

Facial Skin Products: How to Choose

When most people think of caring for skin, they automatically think of their face. There are tons of products on the market meant to be applied to the face in order to make the skin healthier and look better. Due to all the products on the market it can be hard for a person to make any decision as to what they should use in order to get the best results. Facial products include cleansers, toners, exfoliators and moisturizers. Facial products are usually classified into categories such as:

- Gender: whether these are for men or women

- Skin type: The products are going to be for oily, dry, combination or normal skin, as well as those for sensitive skin.

- Age: Many products are geared towards a specific age group

- Disorders of the skin: products that are meant to treat disorders such as acne.

With this being said, a good starting point for finding the best facial product for your skin is to determine what type of skin that you have. Skin types are going to change with age and may even change due to the environment in which you are. Thus, you may have to make changes to your facial products every once in a while.

Products are available in creams, lotions, masks, gels and the like. Many people ask what the best form of the facial product is for them, and this is really depending on what the person wants. The best form is what you are most comfortable with using. All of these products are going to work differently for each person out there. The best way to determine what to use is to simply try out a few products.

You should also consider what state your skin is in when choosing a facial skin product. If you have any sort of problem with your skin, you need to choose a product that is for this problem. Along with choosing the correct facial skin product for you, you also need to make sure that you are using this as it should be used. Complications can come from not using the product as it is designed.

Skin Products: Whats the Best

The main question that people ask is just what is the best skin product on the market. To be honest, there really is no product that is considered the best. Every person is going to have something that works for him or her, yet it may not work for everyone else. The idea is to find the product that is going to work best for the type of skin that you have. Whether this is dry skin, oily skin, normal skin or sensitive skin. All of the products on the market are usually geared at one or a combination of a few of these skin types.

In order to find the best skin product for you, you need to look at the ingredients on the product. All products have two types of ingredients which are active and inactive. The active ingredients work on the skin, while the inactive ingredients are meant to deliver the active ingredients. You should also consider the way in which this is applied to the skin, and how many times you use the product.

There are environmental factors that are going to affect how well a skin product works for you which must be taken into consideration when looking at the best skin care product for you. For those who want the best skin care product for them, consider the following tips to ensure that you are getting the most out of your product:

1. Always cleanse your skin before doing anything else to your skin

2. Always remove your makeup with makeup remover

3. Always use your best skin product first before applying something else as these can cancel out the active ingredients in one another

4. Always apply products on skin that is warm and damp

5. Do not over exfoliate as this can cause skin damage

You will find that as the weather changes you will need to change the products that are using as the skin changes with the weather. You are not going to find the best skin product for you overnight, you will have to stick with the product for a week or two in order to determine whether this is effective for you or not.

Skin Care: The Natural Way

Those who prescribe to the natural skin care phase are all about using products that are free from chemicals and all natural. The idea behind the use of these types of products is that the person can get the skin to basically balance itself out without the use of chemicals that many other products contain. There are several people who simply believe that following good habits is going to help the person's skin to balance itself out naturally. There are several advocates of this approach. Whether or not this approach is for you, is really up to the individual. However, in an effort to understand natural skin care, there are several aspects that a person must take in mind when wanting to adopt this type of skin care system.

One of the cardinal rules of natural skin care is to drink lots of water. Those who want to do this right will find that they have to drink at least eight glasses of water each day. Water is known for helping to flush toxins that are in the body. It is thought that the more toxins that are flushed from the body the better the body functions, and this also includes the better the skin will look. It is a good idea for everyone to follow this rule as it does help the organs within the body to function better.

Being clean is also a part of natural skin care. This involves taking showers everyday, wearing clean clothes each day and sleeping on a pillow and sheets that are clean. The idea is that the oils in the body are not going to be a problem, once the person is not submerging their skin repeatedly into the same oils that the skin will balance itself out.

Those who are strong proponents of this type of skin care emphasize that daily exercise is a necessity. The blood flow is increased when the person increases, which helps to rid the body of the toxins that may be in, as well as serving as a way to keep the person healthy all the way around. Stress is also something that exercise beats, which has been linked to many skin conditions a person could have.

The way in which the person eats also needs to be healthy. This will mean avoiding foods that are very oily, which can transfer to the skin being oilier. In addition, oily foods have been known to cause acne or to further worsen the acne the person is dealing with. Vegetables and raw fruits are a great addition to any diet, and are known for helping the body to rid it of toxins, thus improving the quality of the person's skin.

Sleeping the recommended amount of hours each night is also great for the skin as this is going to help the person to deal with stress better. In addition, sleeping can improve the elasticity in the skin, which means having to deal with less wrinkles and sagging skin as the person ages.

The person should also consider how they deal with stress. The better the person deals with stress can help their skin out tremendously. Stress does cause damage to the body. Stress relievers can include drinking the right amount of water, getting the recommended amount of sleep and exercising. However, the person needs to find something that is going to help them deal with stress, whether this is a relaxing bath, listening to their favorite music or playing a sport. For those who are interested, yoga is a great way to get fit and to beat the stress the person is under. In fact, there are more and more people each day who are diving into yoga for this particular reason.

The exposure the person gets when it comes to the sun can also be a way to deal with their skin naturally. This means avoiding the sun by wearing the right clothing or using hats or umbrellas to shield your skin. Sunscreen is a must have for anyone who wants to protect their skin.

There are several products on the market that are natural, as well as several home remedy methods that have proven to be great in helping the skin to be as good as possible. These types of products are relatively inexpensive and they are easy for a person to put into their daily skin routine. Commercial products are usually those like lavender oil, aloe vera and the like, all of which do not have any side effects.

Skin Care: The Organic Way

Organic skin care is something that many people are interested in as it is a means to achieve the skin the person wants without using artificial ways in which to achieve this. Most of these people have the idea that if this can be done naturally, why would the person use something that is not found in nature. This is considered to be the most natural way in which a person can deal with their skin and improve it. Organic skin care has been around for centuries and is the first way in which mankind was able to help their skin's appearance. The good news is that this type of skin care is not going to hurt the skin with unwanted side effects, and it is considered to be an inexpensive method to use. Those who use organic skin care can help their skin with any disorder and maintain the appearance of the skin that they have always wanted.

The use of organic vegetables and fruits is the most popular way in which a person can help their skin. For example, many people use cucumber in their organic routine, along with apple, turmeric, ginger and papaya, just to name a few of the major ingredients people use. You are going to find that any book out there is going to mention these types of fruits and vegetables as ways to help the skin. However, it is up to you to find which is going to work best for your skin type and to deal with the problems that you may be having. It is imperative that you only use fresh vegetables and fruits on the skin as the types that are a bit older and may be closer to rotting are not going to provide the benefits that fresh do.

Milk is one of those products that have been used for centuries in cleansing the skin. There are many commercial products that utilize milk in order to get the skin cleaner. Those who are interested in a good cleaner will find that ground oatmeal combined with milk can make a fantastic cleanser. In fact, those who have oily skin will find that the oatmeal is going to absorb the oil in the skin. This can be combined with honey, fruits, or even egg in order to get even more beneficial results.

Wheat germ is also a very popular organic skin product. This product has a ton of Vitamin E in it and is known as a great exfoliator for the skin, while also providing a lot of moisture for the skin. Wheat germ is often used as a main ingredient in facial masks and is for normal to dry skin types. This product can be found in an oil format, which is even better for those with dry skin. For those who are looking for an exfoliating product will find that sour cream and yogurt are also popular to use in these circumstances.

Honey that is organic is also great for the skin as it helps the skin to hold in its natural moisture, while also providing the person with a great glow to their skin. Those who are interested in a toner product will find that rose water or lavender water are both known for their ability to tone the skin great.

The whole idea of organic skin care is to use a combination of organic materials that are going to help the skin. These products are going to compliment each other in providing the type of results the person is yearning for. Those who use this method need to realize that this is something that will take time to perfect, but once the person gets there they are going to have amazing looking skin.

Skin Care: The Herbal Way

Skin care is not something that has popped up overnight. For centuries people have always looked for ways to improve the appearance of their skin. During ancient times, the use of herbs was common for those who wanted perfect skin. However, as science progressed more people turned to the use of artificial ingredients that were manufactured in a lab. Herbal skin care is not as common as it once was, and many people tend to forget that they have this option for their skin. There are two main culprits for the end of herbal care for the skin and these are:

- The general population becoming lazier and wanting a product that is going to do it all in the less amount of time that is possible.

- The skin care market has become more commercialized with several companies competing for consumers.

With this being said, herbal skin care products are even being commercialized now as one of the safer ways in which a person can take care for their skin. The problem is that the herbal products on the consumer market do have preservatives in them to give the product a longer shelf life. This does mean that they are not as effective as the use of the old recipe. Though more people are adopting the idea of using herbal remedies for their skin, many people are still not wanting to make these products on their own and they are turning to the commercial products on the market that boast herbs.

There are several herbs on the commercial market that are making up the products that are advertising themselves as being herbal in nature. These include:

- Aloe vera which is extracted form the aloe plant. This is an ingredient that helps to soothe the skin, while also helping to aid in the healing of cuts and the like.

- There are many herbs that are used to help with the cleansing of the skin. These products include chamomile, lime flowers, dandelion and rosemary. These are often combined with teas to help with the healing properties.

- There are several herbs that provide antiseptic relief such as marigold, thyme, lavender and fennel.

- Toners that are herbal are lavender water or rose water.

- To counteract the UV damage skin may have, the use of tea extracts are being used.

- Oils are a huge in the herbal skin care market, These oils can be tea tree oil, borage oil, lavender oil and primrose oil, just to name a few of the most Polaris. There are also many fruits that are used in order to moisturize the skin.

There are also homeopathic and aromatherapies that are considered herbal care that are becoming more common for those who are seeking a less invasive form of skin care. Herbal skin care is going to provide nourishment to the skin, but the care is also known for helping with problem skin such as those who have psoriasis or eczema. These products that are herbal do not have any side effects, which is one of the main reasons that people are opting to use these instead of commercial grade products. In addition, they can easily be made at home with the right ingredients. However, with this being said, that does not mean that a person will get away from the use of commercial products. There are certain skin problems that must be dealt with using these commercial products. If the dermatologist recommends a synthetic product, it best to heed their advice in order to get the flawless skin you are wanting.

Natural Products: Better for Skin?

There are many people who are very intrigued as to what skin products they use on their skin. These people are looking for results that are the least invasive to their skin. Thus, there are tons of people who will only use natural skin care products. They few all commercial grade products as being harmful to their skin. The main question that people ask is if natural products are better for the skin? Are natural skin products going to treat all skin problems that people have? And if the commercial products are so harmful, how are they not banned from being sold to the consumer market?

These are all great questions, and depending on who is asked, there is going to be various answers given. It is important to keep in mind that those who claim they only use natural skin care products are more than likely not aware that those natural products on the market still contain preservatives and chemicals in order to make the product last for much longer. It is almost impossible to find a product that is one hundred percent natural. And those that are claiming to be are more than likely going to cost much more than any other product on the market, and will have to purchased more since the more natural a product, the less time the product will last until it goes bad.

The idea that the natural products are not going to harm the skin is wrong. There are skin types that are going to be harmed by a natural product just as if it were a synthetic product. The idea is to use a product that is catering towards your skin type, whether this is natural or not. Thus, keep an open mind when it comes to using skin products, as you want the one that is going to benefit your skin the most.

When looking at a product that is all natural, there are three factors in which a person must take into consideration:

1. What your skin type is, whether it is normal, dry, sensitive, and oily or a combination type.

2. The type of climate that you are in, such as being hot and humid or dry and cold. The more hot and humid climates are going to want to opt for natural products that are oil free, while those in colder and dry climates may need the extra oil that a product with oil can offer.

3. How the product is applied, since if you do not apply this correctly, you may as well not use any product at all.

Keep in mind that you can make your own natural products to use on your skin with the recipes that can easily be found online or through various books. Most of these recipes are going to utilize fruits and vegetables that are organic, as well as herbal oils.

Though you may be ready to go with an all natural skin care routine, keep in mind that you still need to exercise, eat right, control your stress, drink water and be clean in order to get your skin to the best it can be. Those who do this in combination with a skin care routine are going to have skin that is beautiful and glowing.

Skin Care: Lotions vs. Creams

There is a battle to the death over which is better, lotion or cream when it comes to the health of the skin of a person. There are tons of products on the market and for every skin problem out there you will find a lotion, gel or cream that is meant to treat it. With all the products on the market, lotions and creams are going to make up the majority of what people buy each period. There will always be a debate as to which better, leaving many consumers wondering which they should be using?

No matter whom you ask, you are going to get a different answer to the question which is better, lotions or creams. The honest answer is that the person will have to make this decision for him or herself. They need to use the product that they are more comfortable in using and which product has the best effect on their skin. Statistically, it seems that creams are preferred over lotions because creams seem to be a little bit easier for people to apply and to get results with. Lotions are a bit greasier, leading many people to think they are not good for their skin. However, when it comes to toners, most people seem to prefer a lotion since there are seldom any creams that are going to double as toners. When it comes to cleansers, lotions and creams are going to be equal in popularity, with more people leaning towards lotions.

Creams are known for being better at keeping the skin more moisturized, thus they are a popular form of moisturizers for the person to use. For this reason, many people who have dry and sensitive skin often opt to use a cream. However, skin creams are not only for those with dry or sensitive skin. There are formulas designed for those with oily or combination skin as well. Due to the ease of application, those who have problem skin and need to apply a product to a certain location, rather than their entire body often use skin creams. Other types of creams that are preferred over lotions are those creams meant for the under eye area or those anti-aging creams.

Whether you decide that a lotion or cream is for you will depend upon what you want personally. However, keep in mind that the cream or lotion is only going to work when the correct skin type is chosen and this is applied correctly.

Skin Care to Take Seriously

Everyone needs to realize that your skin is something that needs to be maintained. Thus, it is essential that the person have a skin care routine. The earlier in life a person starts their skin care routine, the happier they are going to be as they age. As you age, the skin becomes weaker, thus the time that you spend on your skin now can make a world of difference later. With this being said, you must be ready to respond to the changes in your skin as you age in order to keep giving your skin what it needs to thrive. Skin care is all about looking at what you need, what you are doing and making changes in order to help with new or developing problems. Not only should you make your skin care decisions based on your age, but also consider the environment in which you live in.

You need to also be aware of the scientific breakthroughs that are happening each day with skin care. The more aware you are of what is happening, the more likely you can reap the benefits from new discoveries. Skin care products are consistently revolving in order to meet the growing needs of the public. Therefore, you should also be up for trying out a new product to see if this is going to be the way to make your skin look healthier and be healthier.

You should always know how to use the products in your skin care arsenal. A few tips to keep in mind are that you should always apply moisturizer when the skin is damp and put this onto the skin in upward motions. You should also remember that you should always remove your makeup before bed, and then follow with your regular cleansing routine to get the best results. You should also strive for skin that is clean and ready to face the world. Also remember that there is a right and wrong way when it comes to how much of the product you utilize. As using too much, is just as bad as using too little.

Always remember to be gentle with your skin. This will mean avoiding the use of harsh detergents or chemicals that could irritate the skin, as well as avoiding exfoliating your skin too much. You should also be mindful of the quality of products you are using as a low quality product can be just as damaging as using too much of something.

With this all in mind, remember that the dermatologist is the professional in which you should turn to. If you have some sort of disorder that you cannot rectify on your own, then it is time to see a professional. Ignoring any problem for any period of time can lead to the person having damage that is beyond repair. This does mean that you should not try to medicate your own skin, such as popping or squeezing pimples, as this can lead to lasting scars.

If you want to be serious about your skin care, then remember this is all about taking the necessary precautions and measure that are meant to prevent problems from occurring. You need to react to any problem you have, while also being proactive to prevent future problems. For those who follow this advice, they will have skin that is healthy and flawless, and before long people will be asking for their secret to having such healthy skin.

We Want Your Feedback on This Book!

Our main purpose is to make sure that our readers get value from the books we publish and that they have a good experience with all of our products. We are always working to improve our books and other products with every revision and update.

Every piece of feedback makes a difference in this process. And we would appreciate yours as well - whether it is good or bad.

Please take one minute to let us know what you thought by following this link:

http://checkmatemg.com/feedbackskincare

www.ingramcontent.com/pod-product-compliance
Lightning Source LLC
Chambersburg PA
CBHW070823290526
45795CB00002B/827